Ketogenic FAT BOMBS RECIPES
Destiny Child

Delicious Low-Carb, High-Fat Sweet & Savory Ketogenic / Paleo Fat Bombs Recipes

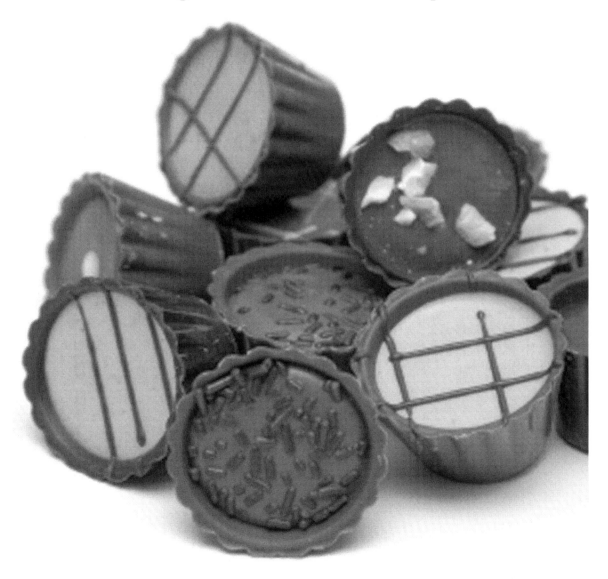

Copyright 2019 by Destiny Child All rights reserved.

This book is copyright protected. This is only for personal use. You cannot amend, distribute, sell, use, quote or paraphrase any part or the content within this book without the consent of the author or copyright owner. Legal action will be pursued if this is breached.

Respective authors own all copyrights not held by the publisher.

The information herein is offered for informational purposes solely, and is universal as so. The presentation of the information is without contract or any type of guaranteed assurance.

The trademarks that are used are without any consent, and the publication of the trademark is without permission or backing by the trademark owner. All trademarks and brands within this book are for clarifying purposes only and are the owned by the owners themselves, not affiliated with this document.

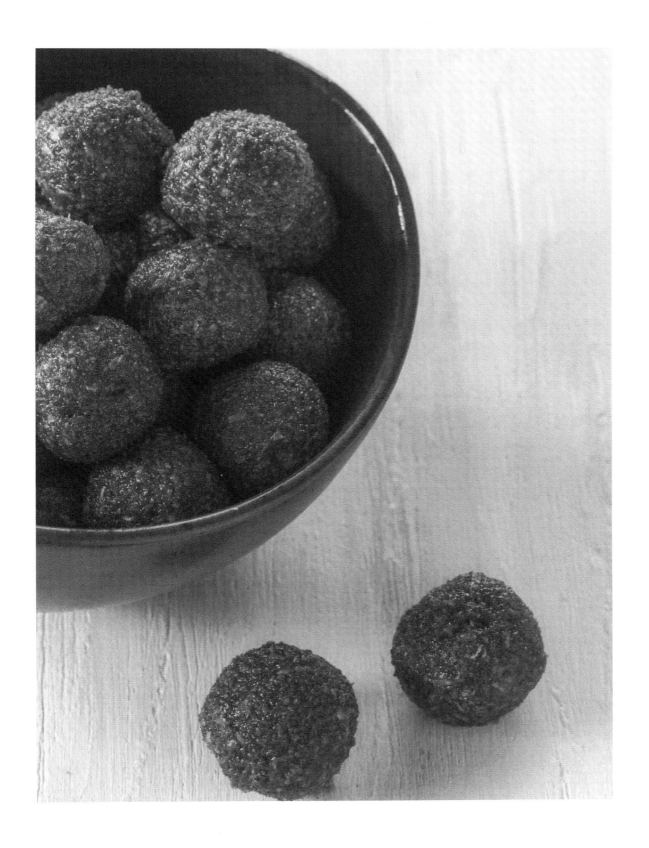

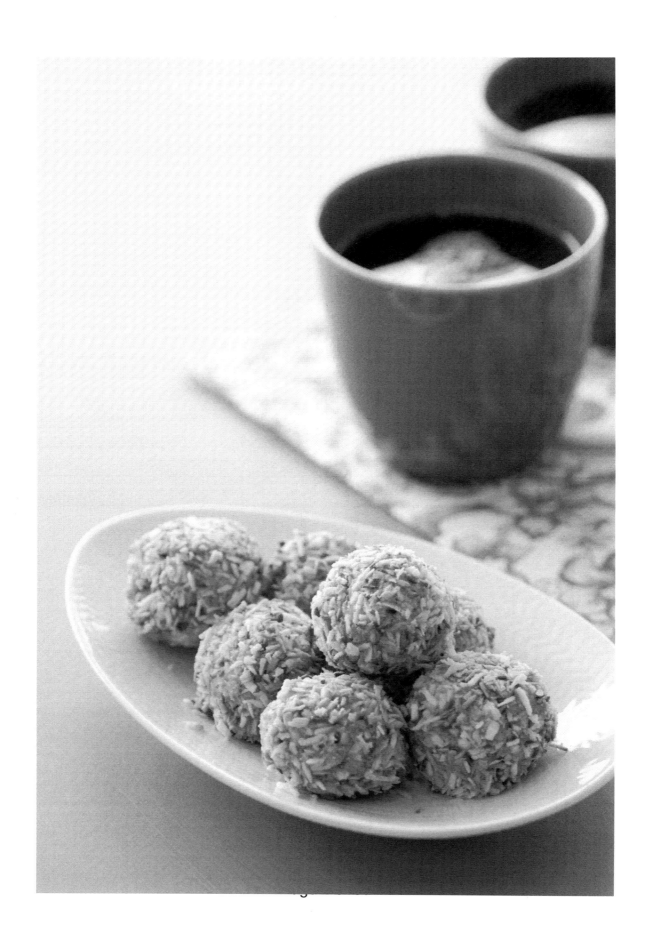

Table of Contents

Ketogenic 1

FAT BOMBS RECIPES 1

Introduction 8

   What is the Ketogenic Diet? 8

   Protect against Obesity 9

   Low-carb Brain Fuel 9

WHAT ARE FAT BOMBS 10

SWEET FAT BOMBS RECIPES 11

   Vanilla Coconut & Pecan Butter 12

   Dairy-free Berries Coconut Cream 13

   Yummy Vanilla Walnut Cinnamon Bars 14

   Delicious Cheesy Coconut Blueberry Cream Bars 16

   Cashew Coconut Almond Bars 18

   Delight Coconut and Cinnamon Muffin 19

   Vanilla Nut Mixed Butter 20

   Healthy Chocolate Layered Coconut Bars 21

   Tasty Shredded Coconut Raspberry Fat Bombs 23

   Great Treat Coconut Candy 24

   Cocoa Minty Chocolate Fat Bombs 25

   Vanilla Coconut Almond Bars 26

   Mini Strawberry Cheesecake 28

   Low-Carb Almond Balls 29

   Stevia Lemon Bombs 30

   Coconut Ginger Bombs 31

Sugar Free Vanilla Lemon 32

Peanut Butter Chocolate Cups 33

Healthy Chocolate & Cayenne Bombs 34

Copycat Sugar-Free Ferrero Rocher 35

Nutmeg Cinnamon Coconut Balls 37

Craving Icy Mocha Fat Bombs 38

Walnut Vanilla Crème Parfaits 39

Delicious Lime Avocado Vanilla Pudding 40

Delight Vanilla Cheesecake Fat Bombs 41

Favorite Coconut Pudding 42

Flavor Matcha Latte Fat Bomb 43

Almond Coconut Cookies 44

Butter Lemon Coconut Cookies 45

Nutmeg Chia Ginger Cookies 47

Yummy Peanut Butter Balls 48

Butter Turmeric Ginger Cookies 49

Quick & Simple Cranberry Fat Bombs 51

No-Bake Mini Lemon Tarts 52

Coconut Blueberry Mug Cake 54

SAVORY FAT BOMBS 56

Bacon Cheese Bars 56

Delicious Garlic Skillet Pepperoni Pizza 57

Healthy Salmon Fat Bombs 59

Avocado bacon balls 60

Keto Sausage Balls 62

Chives Tomato Cheesy Bites 63

Delicious Jalapeno Cheesy Bacon Popper 64

Yummy Bacon & Green Onions 65

Delightful Pecan Bacon Chocolate Bark 66

Healthy Bacon Avocado Bombs 68

Olive Parmesan Pesto Dip 69

Garlic Butter Bacon & Pecan Rolls 70

Cheddar Scallions Creamy Bacon Dip 71

Supreme Sausage Pizza Bomb 72

Garlic Coconut Parmesan Chips 73

Dijon Mustard Cashew Sausage Ham 74

Egg & Cheesy Fat Bombs 75

Delicious Olive Pesto Bombs 76

Prosciutto Avocado Fat Bombs 77

Cheesy Garlic & Lemon Fat Bombs 78

Thick Cut Bacon Cheese Sticks 79

Conclusion 80

Introduction

I want to thank you and congratulate you for purchased the book, "KETOGENIC FATBOMBS RECIPES: Delicious Low-Carb, High-Fat Sweet & Savory Ketogenic / Paleo Fat Bombs Recipes"

What is the Ketogenic Diet?

Our body needs energy from proteins, fats and carbohydrates in order to function properly. Since we've had many years of conditioning our bodies towards a high-carb low-fat diet for our health, our bodies have become highly dependent on glucose from carbohydrates for the majority of our daily energy. It gets to the point where out body isn't breaking down fat at all, and is only sourcing its energy from glucose. Only when glucose and the carb source for it runs out will the fat burning process start up again. The ketogenic diet is great for pushing our body into this ketosis state.

This diet, sometimes called the keto diet, turns your body into an efficient fat-burning machine. This diet has been scientifically supported by nutrition experts and is filled with all sorts of benefits:

- *Increased mental focus*
- *Lowered levels of excess inflammation in the body*
- *Appetite control*
- *Using of natural body fat as main source of fuel*
- *Better stability in blood glucose levels*
- *Lowers risk and elimination of heartburn symptoms*
- *Weight loss*

If you stick to the ketogenic diet, these effects are only the tip of the iceberg. There is plenty more to discover with this diet. The Ketogenic diet has a high-fat, low-carb and moderate protein content with each of the featured meals.

It works like this: If we limit our body's carb source in our diet, our body is encouraged to burn fats for energy in its place in a process called ketosis.

Protect against Obesity

Other studies have shown significant improvements in the BMI of patients that are overweight or obese when aided by ketogenic meals. Millions of people are afflicted with obesity, a condition reaching across the world, and with the help of the ketogenic diet, only a small amount of exercise is needed to lose that extra baggage!

Cholesterol and blood sugar benefit from taking food from the ketogenic diet. However, blood triglyceride levels – which are an important factor in weight gain – is also benefited. What's more, once patients quit the diet and returned to eating normally, they saw a rapid increase in weight again, so perseverance is key.

Low-carb Brain Fuel

An important benefit of the ketogenic diet is the increased mental clarity and focus. By boosting ketone circulation throughout the body, your brain gets better energy sources pumped to it, and this thus reduces the incidence of developing brain and neurological condition.

Control your blood glucose levels in order to encourage fat loss.

The ketogenic diet's main objective is to induce a state of ketosis in the body. Removing most sources of carbohydrate and restricting blood glucose levels will prevent our body from using it as a prime fuel source for energy. Fats will instead be used as the main energy source, and you'll no longer have to worry so much about your weight and focus on feeding your mind and body healthily.

Thanks again for purchasing this book. I hope you enjoy it!

WHAT ARE FAT BOMBS

"Fat bombs" are one part of the Ketogenic diet, but decidedly a fun part! They're often made from a selection of fat-filled ingredients such as coconut oil, nuts, butter and seeds. They're designed specifically for those who are following the ketogenic diet.

As you know, those who are on the diet commit to a high-fat low-carb diet which allows for ketosis state to be encouraged in the body.

Since fat is the main source of fuel in the ketogenic diet, and carbs/sugar is secondary, Fat Bombs are useful for filling this quota. They can be either sweet or savoury.

Fat bombs are, as per the name, high in fat. However, remember that there are good fats and bad fats. The kinds that make up fat bombs are good fats. Similar to the paleo diet, these healthy fats can help to reduce the excess inflammation in your body. Ketogenic fat bombs, for the most part, use coconut derived fats as an ingredient. Coconut oils also solidify into a solid form when kept in the fridge too, which makes these fat bombs both tidy and convenient.

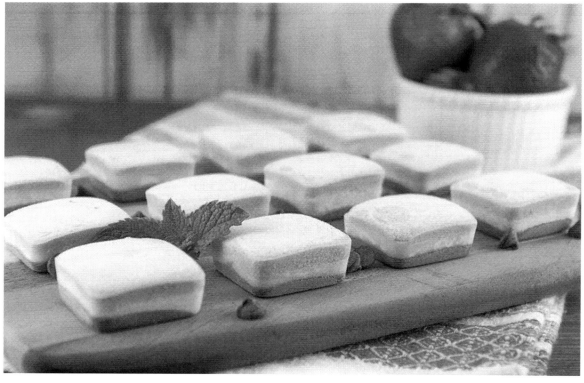

SWEET FAT BOMBS RECIPES

There are 3 basic ingredients to every fat bomb recipe:

 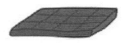 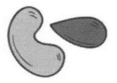

HEALTHY FATS   **FLAVORING**   **TEXTURE**

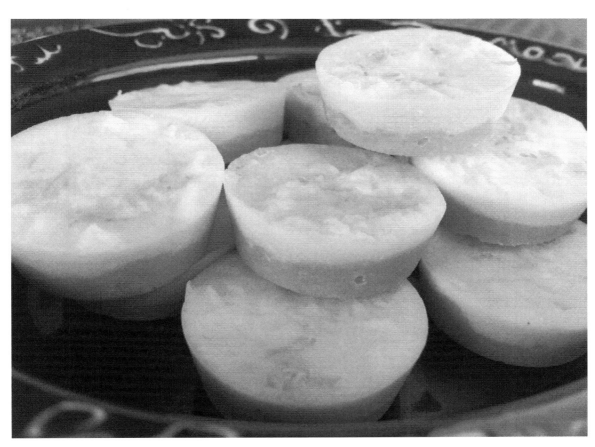

Vanilla Coconut & Pecan Butter

Prep Time: 5 Minutes

Cook Time: 20 Minutes

Serves: 8

Ingredients:

- 2 Cups Unsweetened Shredded Coconut

- 1 Cup Pecan Nuts

- 1 Teaspoon Vanilla Extract

- ½ Teaspoon Cinnamon

- ½ Teaspoon Salt

Directions:

1. Place your pecan nuts and shredded coconut into the food processor, and process it until it's finely chopped.

2. Add your vanilla extract, cinnamon and salt and keep processing it for thirty to sixty seconds. Scrape the sides, and then pulse more. Process until you get the desired consistency, and then store it at room temperature.

Nutritional Information:

Calories: 154

Total Fat: 11.6 g

Total Carbs: 4.5 g

Protein: 5 g

Dairy-free Berries Coconut Cream

Prep Time: 5 Minutes

12 hours freezing

Serves: 2

Ingredients:

- *1 can coconut milk, unsweetened, full-fat*
- *Berries of choice*

Optional:

- *Dark chocolate shavings*
- *Dash of vanilla*

Directions:

1. Refrigerate the coconut milk for at least 12 hours to overnight.

2. Scoop out the coconut cream, leaving the water.

3. Whip the coconut cream with a hand mixer for about 2-3 minutes.

4. Add the berries (blueberries and strawberries are perfect for this).

5. Top with chocolate shavings and dash of vanilla, if desired.

Nutritional Information

Calories: 450

Total Fat: 25.9 g;

Carbohydrates: 14.1 g;

Protein: 4.9 g;

Yummy Vanilla Walnut Cinnamon Bars

Prep Time: 15 Minutes

20 minutes freezing

Serves: 12

Ingredients:

For the chocolate bottom layer:

- *4 tablespoons coconut oil*
- *4 tablespoons cocoa powder*
- *1 teaspoon vanilla extract*
- *3 teaspoons stevia or Splenda*
- *1/4 cup walnuts, chopped*

For the peanut butter top layer:

- *1/2 cup peanut butter*
- *1 tablespoon cinnamon*
- *Pinch sea salt*

Directions:

1.Microwave the coconut oil for about 45 seconds or until melted.

2.Stir in the sweetener, cocoa, and vanilla, mixing well until the mixture is smooth.

3.Fold in the chopped walnuts.

4.Pour the mixture into a dish or pan. Spread evenly.

5. Mix the peanut butter top layer ingredients. Gently pour over the chocolate mixture layer.

6. Sprinkle with sea salt.

7. Freeze for about 20 minutes or until set.

8. Slice into 12 equal-sized pieces. Serve.

Nutritional Information

Calories: 125

Total Fat: 11.7 g;

Carbohydrates: 4.1 g

Protein: 3.7 g

Delicious Cheesy Coconut Blueberry Cream Bars

Prep Time: 25 Minutes

1 hour freezing

Serves: 20

Ingredients:

- *1 cup blueberries, crushed whole or pureed*

- *8 ounces unsalted butter*

- *4 ounces Neufchatel or cream cheese, softened*

- *1/4 cup coconut cream*

- *3/4 cup coconut oil*

- *Splenda or any low-carb sweetener, to taste*

Directions:

For whole berries version:

1.Pour the crushed blueberries into the bottom of the pan or dish.

2.In a saucepan, melt the coconut oil and butter over low heat.

3.Remove from the heat. Allow to cool for 5 minutes.

4.Add the remaining ingredients into the melted coconut oil-butter mixture. With a hand blender or whisk, whip the ingredients together, adding sweetener little by little.

5.Pour the mixture over the blueberries in the pan.

6.Place the pan in the freezer. Freeze for about 1 hour or until set.

7.Slice into 20 equal-sized pieces. Top with a few whole blueberries. Serve.

For pureed version:

1.Place the pureed blueberries, Neufchatel cheese, and coconut cream in a blender or food processor. Puree until the mixture is smooth.

2.In a saucepan, melt the coconut oil and butter over low heat.

3.Remove from the heat. Allow to cool for 5 minutes.

4.Add the sweetener. Pour the melted coconut oil-butter into the blender or food processor. Puree again until smooth.

5.Pour the pureed mixture into molds, cupcake liners, or tins.

6.Freeze for about 1 hour or until the mixture is firm.

Nutritional Information

Calories: 178

Total Fat: 19.5 g;

Carbohydrates: 1.5 g;

Protein: 0.8 g;

Cashew Coconut Almond Bars

Prep Time: 5 Minutes

Cook Time: 15 Minutes

Serves: 8

Ingredients:

- 1 cup almond flour
- 1/4 cup butter
- 1/2 cup sugar free maple
- 1 teaspoon cinnamon
- 1 pinch Salt
- 1/2 cup cashews, chopped
- 1 cup shredded coconut

Directions:

1. In a bowl, add all ingredients and mix well.

2. Spread in a large platter evenly and freeze for 3 hours.

3. Cut in the form of bars and serve.

Nutritional Information

Calories: 205

Total Fat: 17g

Carbohydrates: 10.1 g

Protein: 4.2 g;

Delight Coconut and Cinnamon Muffin

Prep Time: 5 Minutes

Cook Time: 15 Minutes

Serves: 12

Ingredients:

- 1 cup almond flour
- 2 tablespoons coconut flour
- 1/2 teaspoon baking powder
- 1/4 teaspoon cinnamon
- 1/2 teaspoon salt
- 1/2 cup Swerve / erythritol
- 2 large eggs
- 4 tablespoons coconut oil
- 1/2 teaspoon vanilla extract
- 1/2 teaspoon almond extract
- 1 tablespoon shredded coconut, organic

Directions: Preheat oven at 355 degrees. In a bowl add all ingredients and mix well until even. Transfer into baking dish and bake for 15 minutes. Cut into bars Serve and enjoy.

Nutritional Information

Calories 103

Total Fat: 9.7 g;

Carbohydrates: 3.0 g;

Protein: 2.8 g;

Vanilla Nut Mixed Butter

Prep Time: 5 Minutes

Total Time: 5 Minutes

Serves: 10

Ingredients:

- 2 Cups Macadamia Nuts

- 8-10 Brazil Nuts

- ½ Teaspoon Vanilla Extract

- ¼ Teaspoon Salt

Directions:

1. Start by placing your Brazil nuts, vanilla, macadamias, and salt in a food processor, and start to blend.

2. Blend until you get your desired consistency. It'll take about two to four minutes depending on how smooth you want it.

You can store at room temperature for about a week, but you can always store it in the fridge for a month.

Nutritional Information:

Calories: 225

Total Fat: 23.6 g

Total Carbs: 4.3 g

Protein: 2.8 g

Healthy Chocolate Layered Coconut Bars

Total Cooking &Prep Time: 30

1 Hour Freezing

Serves: 12

Ingredients:

For the coconut bottom layer:

- *2 cups shredded coconut, unsweetened*

- *2 drops liquid stevia*

- *1/3 cup coconut oil, virgin, melted*

For the chocolate top layer:

- *3 squares Baker's chocolate, unsweetened (1 Baker's unsweetened chocolate bar is 1 ounce)*

- *2 drops liquid stevia (about 1 teaspoon stevia powder)*

- *1 tablespoon coconut oil*

Directions:

For the coconut bottom layer:

1.Into a food processor, using the S-blade, place the entire ingredients.

2.Process until the mixture forms into dough that falls away from the sides. Scrape down the sides when needed.

3.When sufficiently processed, put the mixture into the bottom of a 9×5-inches silicone loaf pan. For a thinner layer, use an 8×8-inches silicone cake pan.

4.Place the pan in the freezer while preparing the chocolate top layer.

For the chocolate top layer:

1.Put the chocolate and the coconut oil in a microwavable bowl. At 50% power, microwave the mixture until the oil and chocolate has melted.

2.When melted, remove bowl from the microwave. Add the sweetener and mix the ingredients until smooth.

3.Pour the melted chocolate over the frozen coconut layer, spreading evenly. Return to the freezer and freeze for about 30 minutes or until the layers are frozen together.

4.When frozen, turn the pan inside out, releasing the frozen mixtures.

5.Cut into 12 equal-sized bars.

Storage:

Place in a Ziploc and keep in the freezer.

Nutritional Information:

Calories: 145

Total Fat: 15.3 g;

Carbohydrates: 5.2 g;

Protein: 1.4 g;

Tasty Shredded Coconut Raspberry Fat Bombs

Prep Time: 5 Minutes

Total Time: 25-30 Minutes

Serves: 12

Ingredients:

- ½ Cup Coconut Butter

- ½ Cup Coconut Oil

- ½ Cup Raspberries, Freeze Dried

- ½ Cup Shredded Coconut, Unsweetened

- ¼ Cup Powdered Sugar Substitute (can be Swerve)

Directions:

1. Take your food processor, and pulse your raspberries until they turn into a fine powder.

2. Combine your coconut oil, coconut butter, shredded coconut, and sweetener in a saucepan, cooking over medium heat and stirring until fully melted.

3. Stir in your raspberry powder after you remove it from heat, and then pour it into your molds. 4. Keep it refrigerated until it's solid.

Nutritional Information:

Calories: 169

Total Fat: 18 g

Total Carbs: 3.2 g

Protein: 0.3 g

Great Treat Coconut Candy

Prep Time: 5 Minutes

Total Time: 15 Minutes

Serves: 10

Ingredients:

- ⅓ Cup Coconut Butter, Softened

- ⅓ Cup Coconut Oil, Melted

- 1 Ounce Shredded Coconut, Unsweetened

- 1 Teaspoon Sugar Substitute

Directions:

Start by mixing all of your ingredients together, and make sure that the sugar substitute is well dissolved.

Pour into silicone molds, and then refrigerate for about an hour.

Nutritional Information:

Calories: 104

Total Fat: 11 g

Total Carbs: 0.8 g

Protein: 0.3 g

Cocoa Minty Chocolate Fat Bombs

Prep Time: 10 Minutes

Total Time: 20 Minutes

Serves: 6

Dairy Free, Nut Free

Ingredients:

- ½ Cup Coconut Oil, Melted

- 2 Tablespoons Cocoa Powder

- 1 Tablespoon Granulated Stevia (or sweetener of choice)

- ½ Teaspoon Peppermint Essence

Directions:

1. Start by melting your coconut oil, and adding your peppermint essence and sweetener.

2. Add cocoa powder to half of the mixture and mix well in another bowl.

3. Pour the chocolate mixture into the silicone molds, and then place them in the fridge. Refrigerate for 5-10 minutes.

3. Make the mint layer by pouring the mint mixture into the silicon molds. Refrigerate for another 5-10 minutes.

4. Pour the last layer of chocolate mixture into the molds. Refrigerate and let harden.

Nutritional Information:

Calories: 161

Total Fat: 18.5 grams

Total Carbs: 1.15 g

Protein: 0.4 grams

Vanilla Coconut Almond Bars

Prep Time: 15 Minutes

Cooking Time: 10 Minutes

4 Hours Freezing

Serves: 24

Ingredients:

- *1/2 cup cocoa butter, melted*
- *1/4 cup pistachio nuts, chopped*
- *1 cup coconut butter*
- *1 cup almond butter*
- *1 cup coconut oil, firm*
- *1 teaspoon coconut milk, chilled*
- *1 tablespoon vanilla extract*
- *1/4 teaspoon almond extract*
- *1/4 cup ghee*
- *2 teaspoons Chai spice*
- *1/4 teaspoon sea salt*

Directions:

1.Grease a 9-inch baking pan and then line it with parchment paper. Set aside.

2.In a small saucepan over low heat, melt the cocoa butter, stirring often. Set aside.

3.Except for the pistachios and cocoa butter, put the rest of the ingredients into a large mixing bowl. With a hand mixer on low speed, mix the ingredients, increasing to high speed, until everything is well-blended, airy, and light.

4.Pour the melted cocoa butter into the mixture. On low speed, continue mixing for about 1-2 minutes.

5.Transfer the mixture into the prepared baking pan. Spread it as evenly as possible.

6.Sprinkle the chopped pistachios over. Refrigerate for about 4-5 hours or until completely set. Freezing it overnight is best.

7.When frozen, cut into 24 equal-sized pieces.

Nutritional Information:

Calories: 227

Total Fat: 23.5 g;

Carbohydrates: 3.2 g;

Protein: 2.6 g;

Mini Strawberry Cheesecake

Prep Time: 5 Minutes

Total Time: 15-20 Minutes

Serves: 8

Ingredients:

- ½ Cup Strawberries, Fresh & Mashed

- ¾ Cup Cream Cheese, Softened

- ¼ Cup Coconut Oil, Softened

- 10-15 Drops Liquid Stevia

- 1 Teaspoon Vanilla Extract

Directions:

1. Start by combining all of the ingredients in a bowl, and mixing with a hand mixer until completely smooth. You can also do this in a high-speed blender.

2. Spoon into mini muffin tins, and place in the freezer. It'll take about two hours to set, and then you can place them in the fridge.

Nutritional Information:

Calories: 129

Total Fat: 13.27 g

Protein: 1.66 g

Total Carbs: 1.55 g

Low-Carb Almond Balls

Prep Time: 15 Minutes

Freeze For: 15 Minutes

Serves: 4

Ingredients:

- 2 tablespoons almond butter
- 2 tablespoons coconut oil, melted
- 2 tablespoons cocoa powder
- 1 tablespoon coconut flour
- Splenda, to taste (or equivalent low-carb sweetener)

Directions:

1. Mix the coconut oil and the cocoa powder.

2. Add the almond butter.

3. Mix until smooth.

4. Add the coconut flour and the sweetener.

5. Form into balls.

6. Place the mixture on wax paper.

7. Freeze for about 5 minutes.

Nutritional Information:

Calories: 128

Total Fat: 12.8 g;

Carbohydrates: 3.7 g;

Protein: 2.3 g;

Stevia Lemon Bombs

Prep Time: 5-10 Minutes

Total Time: 35-45 Minutes

Serves: 16

Ingredients:

- ¾ Cup Coconut Butter, Softened

- ¼ Cup Virgin Coconut Oil, Softened

- 2 Tablespoons Lemon Extract

- ¼ Tablespoon Lemon Zest

- 15-20 Drops Stevia Extract

Directions:

1. Start by mixing your coconut butter and coconut oil until blended.

2. Add lemon extract, lemon zest and liquid sweetener and stir. Make sure that it's completely blended.

3. Take mini muffin paper cups, and put a tablespoon of the mixture in each one before placing them in the fridge.

4. Refrigerate them until they're solid. This can take anywhere from thirty minutes to an hour depending on where you place them and what temperature your fridge is set at. Pop one out when you want to eat it.

Nutritional Information:

Calories: 118; Total Fat: 13.6 g Carbs: 0.15 g ;Protein: 0.01 g

Coconut Ginger Bombs

Prep Time: 5 Minutes

Total Time: 20 Minutes

Serves: 10

Ingredients:

- *⅓ Cup Coconut Butter, Softened*

- *⅓ Cup Coconut Oil, Softened*

- *2 Tablespoons Shredded Coconut, Unsweetened*

- *1 Teaspoon Powdered Sweetener*

- *1 Teaspoon Ginger Powder*

Directions:

1. Mix all of your ingredients, and then pour them into a jug. Make sure that you dissolve the sweetener.

2. Once it's dissolved, pour the mixture in silicon molds, and then refrigerate for at least 10 minutes.

Nutritional Information:

Calories: 120

Total Fat: 12.8 g

Protein: 0.5 g

Total Carbs: 2.2 g

Sugar Free Vanilla Lemon

Prep Time: 15 Minutes

Freezing Time: 30 Minutes

Serves: 12

Ingredients:

- *1/2 cup coconut butter, softened*
- *1/2 cup coconut oil, extra-virgin, softened*
- *Juice and zest of 1 lemon*
- *Seeds from 1/2 of a vanilla bean*

Directions:

1.Into a spouted cup, whisk all of the ingredients together.

For discs:

1.Line a 12-mold mini cupcake pan with parchment paper liners.

2.Pour the coconut butter mixture into the liners, dividing evenly.

3.Refrigerate for about 30 minutes or until the mixture is firm.

4.If desired, garnish with fresh lemon zest.

For mini cubes:

1.Line a loaf pan with parchment paper.

2.Pour the coconut butter into the pan.

3.Refrigerate for about 30 minutes or until the mixture is firm.

4.Cut into 1/2-inch cubes. Plate them with toothpicks.

5.If desired, garnish with fresh lemon zest.

Nutritional Information: Calories: 105 ;Total Fat: 11.3 g; ;Carbohydrates: 1.5 g; ;Protein: 0.3 g;

Peanut Butter Chocolate Cups

Prep Time: 15 Minutes

Cook Time: 10 Minutes

Freezing Time: 30 Minutes

Serves: 12

Ingredients:

- *3/4 cup coconut oil*
- *1/4 cup cocoa powder*
- *1/4 cup peanut butter*
- *1 teaspoon coconut oil*
- *30 drops liquid stevia, to taste*

Directions:

1.Heat the 3/4 cup coconut oil until melted. When melted, divide into 3 bowls.

2.In one bowl of oil, stir in the cocoa powder until completely dissolved. Add about 6 drops of liquid stevia. Stir to mix.

3.In another bowl of oil, add the peanut butter. Blend until smooth. Add 6 drops of liquid stevia.

4.In the last bowl, add the 1 teaspoon coconut oil. Add the remaining liquid stevia.

5.Divide the chocolate mixture into 12 small cups. Refrigerate for about 10 minutes or until firm.

6.When chocolate mix is firm, divide the peanut butter mixture over the chocolate mixture. Return to the fridge until set. When firm, divide the coconut oil mixture over the hard peanut butter layer. Chill until firm and ready to serve.

Nutritional Info : Calories: 153 ;Total Fat: 16.6 g; ;Carbohydrates: 2.1 g; ;Protein: 1.7 g;

Healthy Chocolate & Cayenne Bombs

Prep Time: 5 Times

Total Time: 15 Minutes

Serves: 12

Ingredients:

- ¼ Cup Coconut Oil

- ¼ Cup Salted Butter, Melted

- ¼ Cup Almond Butter

- 2 Tablespoons Cocoa Powder

- 3 Teaspoons Liquid Sweetener

- ¼ Teaspoon Cayenne Pepper

Directions:

1. Melt coconut oil and butter in a saucepan over low heat.

2. Mix all of your ingredients together in a mixing bowl, and then pour them into silicon molds of your choice.

2. Freeze for at least 30 minutes before eating.

Nutritional Information:

Total Carbs: 2.85 g

Protein: 1.42 g

Total Fat: 10.14 g

Calories: 102

Copycat Sugar-Free Ferrero Rocher

Prep Time: 10 Minutes

Freezing Time: 1-2 Hours

Serves: 12

Ingredients:

For the balls:

- *1/2 cup homemade Nutella, recipe follows in Other Ketogenic Desserts*

- *12 hazelnuts*

For the coating:

- *2 ounces chocolate bar, sugar-free*

- *1/4 cup hazelnuts, chopped*

Directions:

1.In a dry skillet, toast the hazelnuts until fragrant. When toasted, remove as much skin as possible. Allow to cool.

2.Refrigerate the homemade Nutella for about 30 minutes. Scoop 1 teaspoon of Nutella, flatten like a mini pancake, and place in a parchment lined baking sheet.

3.Top the flattened Nutella with 1 hazelnut. Top with another 1 teaspoon flattened Nutella. Mold into ball shape. Make 12 balls. Refrigerate.

4.Melt the chocolate bar. When melted, stir in the chopped nuts. Mix well.

5. Line a baking sheet with parchment paper. Place a wire rack on the baking sheet.

6. Take 1 Nutella ball. Hold the ball with fork, dip in the chocolate coating, and take out, removing excess. Place the coated balls in the prepared wire rack. Repeat with the remaining ingredients.

7. Refrigerate until the coating is hard.

8. Individually wrap each ball with foil, if desired. Store in an airtight container and keep refrigerated until ready to serve.

Nutritional Information:

Calories: 161

Total Fat: 15.8 g;

Carbohydrates: 5.4 g;

Protein: 3.9 g;

Nutmeg Cinnamon Coconut Balls

Prep Time: 90 Minutes

Cook Time: 5 Minutes

Serves: 10

Ingredients:

- *1 cup coconut butter (or almond butter)*
- *1 cup coconut milk (canned, full fat)*
- *1 cup coconut, shredded*
- *1 teaspoon stevia powder extract (or to taste)*
- *1 teaspoon vanilla extract (gluten-free)*
- *1/2 teaspoon cinnamon*
- *1/2 teaspoon nutmeg*

Directions:

1.Put a few inches of water into a saucepan. Place a glass bowl over, creating a double boiler.

2.Except for the shredded coconut, put all of the ingredients into the bowl. Heat over medium heat, mixing the ingredients until melted. Combine well.

3.Place the bowl in the fridge, cooling the mixture for about 30 minutes until it's hard enough to roll into balls.

4.Roll into 1-inch ball and then roll into shredded coconut.

5.Place the balls on a plate and then refrigerate for about 1 hour.

6.Keep refrigerated.

Nutritional Information:

Calories: 142 ;Total Fat: 13.8 g;Carbohydrates: 5.3 g; ;Protein: 1.4 g;

Craving Icy Mocha Fat Bombs

Prep Time: 10 Minutes

Total Time: 1 Hour 10 Minutes

Serves: 12

Ingredients:

- 8.5 Ounces Cream Cheese

- 2 Tablespoons Powdered Sweetener

- 2 Tablespoons Cocoa Powder, Unsweetened

- ¼ Cup Strong Coffee, Chilled

- 2.5 Ounces Dark Chocolate, Melted

- 1 Ounce Cocoa Butter, Melted

Directions:

1. Start by adding your coffee, cream cheese, cocoa powder, and sweetener in a blender, and pulse until it's completely smooth.

2. Roll about two tablespoons of the mixture into small bowls, putting them on a baking sheet lined with parchment paper. This recipe should make twelve.

3. Now, blend the melted dark chocolate and cocoa butter until smooth.

4. Roll your balls in the chocolate coating and place them back on the tray.

5. Freeze them for 1 hour or until set.

Nutritional Info: Carbs: 6.52 g ;Protein: 2.4 g ;Fat: 9.9 grams ;Calories: 120

Walnut Vanilla Crème Parfaits

Prep Time: 10 Minutes

Serves: 4

Ingredients:

- *1 can (398 ml) coconut milk, full-fat, chilled*
- *10 drops liquid stevia (or 1 packet stevia powder)*
- *1 teaspoon vanilla extract, pure, alcohol-free preferred*
- *6 ounces berries, fresh*
- *3 ounces walnuts, chopped*

Optional:

Ground cinnamon

Directions:

1.In the bowl of a stand mixer, add the coconut milk, vanilla extract, and stevia. Whip with the whisk attachment for about 30 seconds until well-mixed. Set aside.

2.In a large bowl, mix the walnuts and the berries. Set aside.

3.Put about 3 spoonfuls of vanilla-coconut crème pudding into 4 jars. Divide 1/2 of the walnut mix between the 4 jars. Spoon a second layer of the vanilla crème pudding over the walnut mixture. Add the remaining walnut mix.

4.Sprinkle each jar with ground cinnamon, if desired.

Nutritional Information:

Calories: 399

Total Fat: 37.5 g;

Carbohydrates: 13.6 g

Protein: 8 g;

Delicious Lime Avocado Vanilla Pudding

Prep Time: 15 Minutes

Serves: 4

Ingredients:

- *1 can (13.5 fl. ounce or 400 ml) coconut milk, organic*
- *1 tablespoon lime juice, freshly squeezed*
- *2 Hass avocados, ripe, peeled, pitted and cut into chunks*
- *2 teaspoons vanilla extract*
- *¾ teaspoon of liquid stevia (or 8 packets stevia powder)*

Directions:

1.Put all of the ingredients into the blender. Close the blender lid.

2.Blend until velvety smooth.

Nutritional Information:

Calories: 445

Total Fat: 43.8 g;

Carbohydrates: 18.8 g;

Protein: 4.2 g;

Delight Vanilla Cheesecake Fat Bombs

Prep Time: 5 Minutes

Total Time: 15 Minutes

Serves: 8

Ingredients:

- 6 Ounces Cream Cheese, Softened

- ½ Cup Heavy Whipping Cream

- 1 ½ Teaspoons Vanilla Extract

- ¼ Cup Erythritol or Other Sugar Substitute

- ¼ Teaspoon Salt

Directions:

1. Add cream cheese, sugar substitute, salt and vanilla extract to a blender. Blend it until smooth.

2. Slowly add the heavy cream.

3. Continue to blend until it's thickened, which will take one to two minutes. It should have a mousse like consistency once you're done.

4. Spoon the mixture into a piping bag and pipe into 8 mini cupcake liners. Chill for one hour until they are set. Keep them refrigerated.

Nutritional Information:

Total Carbs: 1.05 g

Protein: 1.66 g

Total Fat: 8.86 g

Calories: 91

Favorite Coconut Pudding

Prep Time: 15 Minutes

Total Time: 15 Minutes

Serves: 4

Ingredients:

- *1 2/3 cups coconut milk*
- *1 tablespoon gelatin*
- *1/2 teaspoon vanilla extract*
- *3 egg yolks*
- *3 tablespoons honey (or ½ teaspoon liquid stevia)*

Directions:

1.In a small bowl, pour the gelatin and 1 tablespoon of the coconut milk. Set aside.

2.In a medium saucepan over medium-low heat, pour the remaining coconut milk and the honey/sweetener.

3.Cook for about 3-5 minutes, stirring occasionally, until the mixture is hot.

4.In a medium bowl, whisking constantly, slowly pour about 1 ladle of the hot milk, add egg yolks.

5.Continuously stirring, pour the egg yolk mixture back into the saucepan.

6.Cook for another 3-4 minutes, or until the mixture is slightly thicker.

7.Add the gelatin mixture into the pot. Whisk to blend well.

8.Pour the mixture into 4 ramekins.

9.Refrigerate for about 2 hours or until the mixture is set.

Nutritional Information:

Calories: 278

Total Fat: 27.2 g;

Carbohydrates: 9.1 g;

Protein: 5.8 g;

Flavor Matcha Latte Fat Bomb

Prep Time: 5 Minutes

Total Time: 10-15 Minutes

Serves: 1

Ingredients:

- *½ Cup Boiling Water*

- *1 Teaspoon Matcha Powder*

- *⅓ Cup Unsweetened Coconut Milk*

- *1 Tablespoon MCT Oil (you can also use extra virgin coconut oil)*

- *3 Drops Liquid Stevia*

Directions:

1. Start by mixing the matcha powder in the boiling water. Make sure it's completely combined.

2. Add MTC oil and whisk it all over again.

3. Use a milk frother to make the coconut milk froth. Next, pour the froth into the glass with your matcha, and sprinkle matcha powder on top.

4. Add the sweetener before serving. (Optional)

Nutritional Information

Total Carbs: 6.29 grams

Protein: 1.8 grams

Total Fat: 202.5 grams

Calories: 211

Almond Coconut Cookies

Prep Time: 5 Minutes

Total Time: 15 Minutes

Serves:8

Ingredients:

- 1 cup almond flour
- 2 eggs
- 1 cup coconut powder
- ½ teaspoon vanilla extract
- ¼ cup butter
- ½ cup cream milk

Directions:

1. Preheat oven to 355 degrees.

2. In a bowl add eggs and beat until smooth.

3. Add butter, almond flour, coconut powder, cream milk, vanilla extract and beat for 1 minute.

4. Transfer into baking dish and bake for 15 minutes.

5. Serve and enjoy.

Nutritional Information:

Calories: 285

Total Fat: 26.2 g;

Carbohydrates: 8.7 g;

Protein: 7.3 g;

Butter Lemon Coconut Cookies

Prep Time: 10 Minutes

Cook Time: 10 Minutes

Serves: 12

Ingredients:

- *3/4 cup coconut butter, softened*
- *2/3 – ¾ cup Swerve / erythritol*
- *1/4 cup cashew butter (I prefer fresh ground, jarred has added oils)*
- *1 teaspoon baking powder (gluten and corn free)*
- *1 tablespoon grated lemon peel*
- *1 egg*
- *1/4 cup FRESH lemon juice, strained (about 1 lemon)*
- *Dash of sea salt*

Directions:

1.Place the softened coconut butter into a blender and food processor. Pulse until the mixture is smooth.

2.Add in the remaining ingredients. Process until well-combined without a trace of lemon peel in the mixture.

3.If your mixture is too soft to mold, refrigerate it for a few minutes to harden.

4.Roll the mixture into 1-inch balls. Place the balls in a parchment lined cookie sheet. Lightly press on the balls to flatten them.

5.Bake at 35oF for about 10-12 minutes or until the edges of the cookies are slightly brown.

6.Allow the cookies to cool in the cookie sheet for a few minutes and then transfer on a cooling rack.

7.Store the cookies in an airtight container. If you want harder cookies, then keep in the refrigerator.

Note:

To make your own coconut butter, blend shredded coconut for about 20 minutes or until you make a paste. You can season the butter with salt, if desired.

Nutritional Information:

Calories: 76

Total Fat: 6.7 g;

Carbohydrates: 5.5 g;

Protein: 2.0 g;

Nutmeg Chia Ginger Cookies

Prep Time: 10 Minutes

Cook Time: 15 Minutes

Serves: 12

Ingredients:

- *1 egg*
- *1/2 teaspoon nutmeg*
- *1/4 cup coconut oil*
- *2 cups whole almonds*
- *2 tablespoons chia seeds*
- *2 tablespoons cinnamon powder*
- *3 tablespoons ginger, freshly grated*
- *Dash of salt*
- *¾ teaspoon liquid stevia*

Directions:

1.Preheat the oven to 350F or 175C.

2.Blend or food process the chia seeds and the almonds.

3.In a large mixing bowl, mix all the ingredients together.

4.Form into small cookies in a parchment paper lined baking tray.

5.Bake for about 15 minutes at 350F.

Nutritional Information: Calories: 148 ;Fat: 12.9 g; Carbohydrates: 6.3 g; Protein: 5.0 g;

Yummy Peanut Butter Balls

Prep Time: 5 Minutes

Freezing Time: 1 Hour

Serves: 8

Ingredients:

- ¼ Cup Peanut Butter

- 2 Tablespoons Butter

- 1 Tablespoon Coconut Oil

- ¼ Cup Peanuts, Crushed

- 3 Drops Liquid Sweetener

Directions:

1. Melt butter, coconut oil and peanut butter in a saucepan over low heat, stirring until combined.

2. Add in your sweetener, and continue to stir.

3. Place the mixture into the freezer for 10 minutes.

3. Form mixture into balls, and then roll them in crushed peanuts.

4. Let chill for at least one hour before serving.

Nutritional Information:

Total Carbs: 2.66 g

Protein: 3.18 g

Total Fat: 9.95 g

Calories: 107

Butter Turmeric Ginger Cookies

Prep Time: 15 Minutes

Cook Time: 10-15 Minutes

Serves: 15

Ingredients:

- *1 cup coconut butter, softened*

- *1 egg*

- *1 teaspoon turmeric powder*

- *1 teaspoon vanilla extract*

- *1/4 cup low-carb granulated sweetener*

- *1/4 teaspoon baking soda*

- *1/4 teaspoon sea salt*

- *1/8 teaspoon black pepper, or more*

- *2 heaping teaspoons ginger, ground*

Directions:

1.Place the egg, coconut butter, and vanilla extract into a food processor. Blend until well- combined.

2.Add the baking soda, sweetener, and all of the spices. Blend again until combined.

3.Form the cookie mixture into 1-inch balls. Place 1 inch apart on a parchment lined cookie sheet. Press each cookie to flatten into cookie shapes. Do not spread too much.

4.Bake at 350F for about 10-15 minutes or until slightly brown.

5.Allow the cookies to cool down a bit on the cookie sheet. They will be fragile fresh out of the oven. When slightly cool, transfer on a cooling rack and allow to cool completely, hardening as they cool.

6.Store in an airtight container.

Notes:

Do not melt the coconut butter completely, just soften it. If the cookie dough mixture does not form into a ball because the butter is too runny, place the mixture in the fridge for a few minutes to make it moldable.

Nutritional Information:

Calories: 44

Total Fat: 3.9 g;

Carbohydrates: 3.6 g;

Protein: 0.8 g;

Quick & Simple Cranberry Fat Bombs

Prep Time: 5 Minutes

Total Time: 15-20 Minutes

Serves: 6

Ingredients:

- 2/3 Cup Cranberries, Dried

- 6 Ounces mascarpone Cheese, Softened

Directions:

1. Chop your cranberries. Make sure that they're chopped fine.

2. Soften your mascarpone cheese, and then blend all ingredients together.

3. Gently spoon the mixture into mini muffin liners and chill for about an hour in the refrigerator before serving.

Nutritional Information:

Total Carbs: 3 g

Protein: 7 g

Total Fat: 10 g

Calories: 125

No-Bake Mini Lemon Tarts

Prep Time: 30 Minutes

Cook Time: 0 Minutes

Serves: 24

Ingredients:

For the crust:

- *4 1/2 tablespoons butter, coconut oil, or ghee, melted*
- *3/4 cup coconut, dried, finely grated*
- *3 tablespoons lemon juice*
- *Low-carb sweetener equivalent to 2 tablespoons sugar*
- *1 cup almond flour, or other nut flour like cashew*
- *1 1/2 teaspoons vanilla extract*
- *Pinch of salt*

For the filling:

- *1 teaspoon vanilla extract, sugar-free*
- *1/2 cup butter, coconut oil, or ghee, softened to room temperature*
- *1/3 cup coconut milk, full fat (or other low-carb milk like almond)*
- *1/3 cup fresh lemon juice*
- *1/4 teaspoon salt*
- *2 teaspoons lemon extract*
- *Grated zest from 2 medium lemons*

- *Low-carb sweetener equivalent to 1/4 cup plus 1 tablespoon sugar*

Directions:

For the crust:

1. *Grease 2 12-cup size mini-muffin pans.*

2. *In a medium mixing bowl, combine all of the crust ingredients until well mixed.*

3. *Roll 2 teaspoons of the crust dough mixture into balls and then press into the prepared tart pans.*

4. *Chill the crusts until ready to fill.*

For the filling:

1. *Put the butter in a bowl. Beat until fluffy. Alternatively, you can blend it in a food processor.*

2. *Add the milk, sweetener, lemon juice, extracts, salt, and zest into the bowl. Beat until the mixture is soft. If using a processor, then blend until smooth.*

3. *Taste test. Add more sweetener or lemon juice as needed.*

To assemble the tarts:

1. *Spoon the filling into the assembled crusts. If desired, garnish with lemon zest.*

2. *Refrigerate until the filling is set.*

Nutritional Information:

Calories: 128

Total Fat: 12.4 g;

Carbohydrates: 3.7 g

Protein: 2.3 g;

Coconut Blueberry Mug Cake

Prep Time: 20 Minutes

Cook Time: 10 Minutes

Serves: 5

Ingredients:

- *1 teaspoon baking soda*
- *1/2 cup coconut milk*
- *1/2 cup frozen wild blueberries*
- *1/2 cup plus 1 teaspoon coconut flour, divided*
- *1/2 teaspoon lemon extract*
- *1/4 cup coconut oil (could also use avocado oil here), melted*
- *1/4 cup Swerve / erythritol sweetener or any low carb sweetener*
- *1/4 teaspoon stevia extract (or equivalent stevia powder)*
- *4 large eggs*
- *Pinch salt*
- *Zest of 1 lemon*

Directions:

1. In a medium mixing bowl, whisk the 1/2 cup coconut flour, baking soda, lemon zest, sweetener, and salt together.

2. Stir in the coconut milk, coconut oil, eggs, stevia extract, and lemon extract.

3. In a small mixing bowl, toss the 1 teaspoon coconut flour and blueberries. Add the coconut flour tossed berries into the batter. Mix gently.

4.Divide the batter between 5 mugs.

5.Cook each mug on high in the microwave for about 1 minute and 30 seconds. You can cook it longer, if desired.

Nutritional Information:

Calories: 303

Total Fat: 28.6 g;

Carbohydrates: 20.5 g;

Protein: 6.6 g;

SAVORY FAT BOMBS

Bacon Cheese Bars

Prep Time: 15 Minutes

Freezing Time: 15 Minutes

Serves: 2

Ingredients:

- *8 ounces Neufchatel cheese, softened*
- *8 slices bacon, cooked, crumbled*
- *4 teaspoons bacon fat*
- *4 tablespoons coconut oil*
- *1/2 cup unsalted butter*
- *1/4 cup sugar-free maple syrup or ¼ cup Swerve / erythritol*

Directions:

1.Set aside 1-2 pieces of crumbled bacon.

2.In a microwavable bowl, combine all of the ingredients together.

3.Put the bowl in the microwave. In 10-second intervals, melt the ingredients.

4.When melted, stir to combine, and then pour into a pan or dish.

5.Freeze for about 15 minutes or until the mixture is set.

6.When frozen, remove from the freezer, sprinkle with the reserved crumbled bacon, slice, and then serve.

Nutritional Information:Calories: 126 ;Total Fat: 11.5 g ;Carbohydrates: 2.6 g; ;Protein: 3.4 g;

Delicious Garlic Skillet Pepperoni Pizza

Prep Time: 10 Minutes

Freezing Time: 20 Minutes

Serves: 4

Ingredients:

- *4 ounces mozzarella cheese, or more to cover the bottom of 10-inch skillet*

- *12 pepperoni slices*

- *1 ounce parmesan cheese*

- *2 tablespoons tomatoes, crushed*

- *1 teaspoon garlic powder*

- *1 teaspoon Italian seasoning or dried basil*

- *1 teaspoon red pepper, crushed*

- *1 teaspoon basil, fresh, torn*

Directions:

1.Heat a small, non-stick skillet over medium heat.

2.Evenly cover the bottom with the mozzarella cheese. This will serve as the crust.

3.With the back of a spoon, lightly spread the tomatoes over the cheese, leaving a border around the edges of the cheese crust.

4.Sprinkle with the garlic powder and the Italian seasoning or dried basil.

5.Arrange the pepperoni on top. Cook until bubbled, sizzling, and the edges of the crust are brown.

6. With a spatula, try lifting the edges. When done, the pizza will lift easily from the pan. If the pizza still sticks, it means it is not yet done. Lift and check frequently.

7. When the pizza lifts up easily, work the spatula slowly and gently underneath, loosening up the entire pizza. Transfer to a cutting board.

8. Lightly sprinkle with parmesan, basil leaves, and red pepper.

9. Cool for about 5 minutes to cool and allow the crust to firm. Cut with a pizza cutter. Transfer to a serving plate.

Nutritional Information:

Calories: 196

Total Fat: 14.3 g;

Carbohydrates: 2.8 g;

Protein: 14.5 g;

Healthy Salmon Fat Bombs

Prep Time: 5 Minutes

Total Time: 10-15 Minutes

Serves: 6

Ingredients:

- ½ Cup Full-Fat Cream Cheese

- 5 Tablespoons Butter

- 1.8 Ounces Smoked Salmon

- 1 Tablespoon Lemon Juice

- 1 ½ Tablespoons Fresh Dill, Chopped

Directions:

1. Start by putting your cream cheese, butter and smoked salmon into a food processor.

2. Add in your dill and lemon juice, pulsing until smooth.

3. Take a tray lined with parchment paper, and then use about 2 ½ tablespoons of the mixture to form each piece. Add more dill for garnish, and allow to firm in the fridge for one to two hours.

Nutritional Information:

Total Carbs: 0.8 g

Proteins: 3.2 g

Total Fat: 15.7 g

Calories: 147

Avocado bacon balls

Total Time: 30 Minutes

Serves: 6

Ingredients:

½ *large avocado (100 g / 3.5 oz)*

¼ *cup butter or ghee*

2 cloves garlic, crushed

1 small chili pepper, finely chopped

½ *small white onion, diced*

1 tbsp fresh lime juice

freshly ground black or cayenne pepper

¼ *tsp salt or more to taste*

1-2 tbsp freshly chopped cilantro

4   slices bacon

Directions:

Preheat the oven to 190 C / 375 F. Line a baking tray with baking paper. Lay the bacon strips out flat on the baking paper, leaving space so they don't overlap. Place the tray in the oven and cook for about 10-15 minutes until golden brown. The time depends on the thickness of the bacon slices. When done, remove from the oven and set aside to cool down.

Halve, deseed and peel the avocado. Place the avocado, butter, chili pepper, crushed garlic, cilantro and lime juice into a bowl and season with salt and pepper. Bacon & Guacamole Fat Bombs

Mash using a potato masher or a fork until well combined. Add the diced onion and mix well. Bacon & Guacamole Fat Bombs

Pour in the bacon grease from the tray where you baked the bacon and mix well. Cover with a foil and place in the fridge for 20-30 minutes.

Crumble the bacon into small pieces and prepare for "breading." Remove the guacamole mixture from the fridge and start creating 6 balls. You can use a spoon or an ice-cream scooper. Roll each ball in the bacon crumbles and place on a tray that will fit in the fridge.

Serve immediately or store in the fridge in an airtight container for up to 5 days.

Nutritional Information:

Total Carbs 2.7g

Protein3.4g

Fat 15.2g

Calories: 156

Keto Sausage Balls

Total Time: 20 Minutes

Serves: 1

Ingredients

- *1 lb. Breakfast Sausage*
- *1 Large Egg*
- *1 Cup Almond Flour*
- *8 Oz Cheddar Cheese*
- *1/4 Cup Grated Parmesan*
- *1 Tbsp Butter (or Coconut Oil)*
- *2 tsp Baking Powder*
- *1/4 tsp Salt*

Directions:

Preheat oven to 350. Add all ingredients in a large mixing bowl and mix until well combined.

Using a cookie scoop and your hands roll sausage mixture into 20-25 sausage balls .Place sausage balls on a cookie sheet

Bake for 16-20 minutes. Store in a sandwich bag or covered bowl in the fridge.

Nutritional Information:

Calories: 124

Total Fat: 11g

Carbohydrates: 1g

Protein: 6g

Chives Tomato Cheesy Bites

Prep Time: 5-10 Minutes

Cook Time: 15-20 Minutes

Serves: 12

Ingredients:

- 3 Ounces Full Fat Cream Cheese

- 12 Cherry Tomatoes

- ¼ Cup Fresh Chives

- Salt to Taste

Directions:

1. Cut a small slice off the top of each cherry tomato and discard seeds and juice.

2. Chop your chives thin, and then mix it with your softened cream cheese and salt.

3. Fill each tomato with flavored cream cheese.

Nutritional Information:

Total Carbs: 1.03 g

Protein: 0.83 g

Total Fat: 2.74 g

Calories: 31

Delicious Jalapeno Cheesy Bacon Popper

Prep Time: 30 Minutes

Cook Time: 10 Minutes

Serves: 1

Ingredients:

- *3 slices bacon*
- *3 ounces cream cheese*
- *1/4 teaspoon onion powder*
- *1/4 teaspoon garlic powder*
- *1/2 teaspoon dried parsley*
- *1 medium jalapeno pepper*
- *Salt and pepper, to taste*

Directions:

1.In a pan, fry the slices of bacon until crisp. Remove the bacon from the pan, keeping the bacon grease for later use. Allow the bacon to cool.

2.De-seed the jalapeno pepper and then dice into small pieces.

3.In a mixing bowl, combine the jalapeno, cream cheese, and spices, seasoning with salt and pepper to taste.

4.Add the bacon fat into the cream cheese. Mix together until a solid mixture is formed.

5.Crumble the crispy bacon and put in a plate.

6.With your hands, roll the cream cheese into balls and then roll each ball into the crumbled bacon.

Nutritional Information: Calories: 614 ;Fat: 53.6 g; Carbohydrates: 5 g; ;Protein: 27.9 g;

Yummy Bacon & Green Onions

Prep Time: 5 Minutes

Total Time: 15 Minutes

Serves: 5

Ingredients:

- 5 Strips Bacon

- 6 Green Onions, Trimmed

- 4 Tablespoons Coconut Oil

- Salt and Pepper to Taste

Directions:

1. Start by wrapping green onions together using a single strip of bacon. Repeat until all of your bacon and green onions are used.

2. Season the wrapped green onions with salt and pepper.

3. Use a frying skillet and heat up coconut oil over medium high heat, frying your wraps until they're slightly browned. This usually takes six to eight minutes.

Nutritional Information:

Total Carbs: 2.82 g

Protein: 1 g

Total Fat: 12.5 g

Calories: 121

Delightful Pecan Bacon Chocolate Bark

Prep. Time: 30 minutes,

Cook Time: 30 minutes

Freezing time; 1 hour

Serves: 20

Ingredients:

For the bacon-pecan crumble:

- *2 tablespoons water*
- *1/2 cup Swerve / erythritol sweetener or any low-carb sweetener equivalent*
- *1 tablespoon butter*
- *1/2 pound bacon, chopped, cooked until crisp*
- *1 1/2 cups pecans, toasted, chopped*

For the chocolate mixture:

- *4 ounces cocoa butter*
- *3/4 cup cocoa powder*
- *2 1/2 ounces unsweetened chocolate*
- *1/4 teaspoon kosher salt*
- *1/2 teaspoon vanilla extract*
- *1/2 cup powdered Swerve / erythritol sweetener, sifted*

Directions:

1.Line a baking sheet with parchment paper.

2.Line a 9×13-inch pan with another parchment paper.

3. In a medium saucepan over medium heat, combine the water and the 1/2 cup Swerve / erythritol sweetener, stirring occasionally. Bring the mixture to a boil and cook for about 7–9 minutes or until the mixture darkens. The mixture will smoke slightly. This will be normal.

4. Remove the saucepan from the heat.

5. Whisk the butter in. Add the bacon and the pecans. Quickly stir to coat and then stir in the salt.

6. Spread the bacon-pecan mixture onto the prepared baking sheet. Allow to cool and then break up into clumps.

7. In a heavy saucepan, melt the chocolate and the butter together until the mixture is smooth.

8. Stir in the powdered sweetener and cocoa powder until the mixture is smooth.

9. Remove from the heat. Stir in the vanilla extract.

10. Stir the crumbled bacon-pecan mixture into the chocolate mixture.

11. Spread the mixture into the prepared 9×13-inch pan.

12. Refrigerate for at least 1 hour or until the mixture is solid. When solid, cut into random-sized pieces.

Nutritional Information

Calories: 246

Total Fat: 22.9 g;

Carbohydrates: 8.8 g;

Protein: 8.3 g;

Healthy Bacon Avocado Bombs

Prep Time: 5 Minutes

Total Time: 15 Minutes

Serves: 8

Ingredients:

- 6 Pecans

- 2 Avocados

- 4 Slices Bacon

Directions:

1. Cook your bacon in a pan over medium-high heat until the bacon is crispy.

2. Take it off of heat, allowing it to cool before crumbling it.

3. Take a bowl and mash your avocados, and then crumble your pecans.

4. Mix all ingredients together, and make round balls using an ice cream scooper.

Nutritional Information:

Total Carbs: 4.74 g

Protein: 2.86 g

Total Fat: 14.27 g

Calories: 151

Olive Parmesan Pesto Dip

Prep Time: 5 Minutes

Total Time: 5 Minutes

Serves: 6

Ingredients:

- 1 Cup Full Fat Cream Cheese

- 2 Tablespoons Basil Pesto

- ½ Cup Parmesan Cheese, Grated

- 8 Olives, Sliced

- Salt and Pepper to Taste

Directions:

1. Mix all of your ingredients together in a mixing bowl.

2. Refrigerate for at least 20 minutes before serving.

Nutritional Information:

Total Carbs: 3.43 g

Protein: 5.42 g

Total Fat: 14.33 g

Calories: 161

Garlic Butter Bacon & Pecan Rolls

Prep Time: 5 Minutes

Total Time: 15 Minutes

Serves: 12

Ingredients:

- 4 Bacon Slices, Cooked

- ½ Cup Pecan Halves, Chopped

- ½ Cup Organic Butter

- 1 Teaspoon Garlic Powder

Directions:

1. Divide your bacon into three parts, and then spread each part with butter.

2. Press your pecan pieces into the butter.

3. Sprinkle with garlic and roll up.

Nutritional Information:

Total Carbs: 0.83 g

Protein: 1.53 g

Total Fat: 14.87 g

Calories: 139

Cheddar Scallions Creamy Bacon Dip

Prep Time: 5-10 Minutes

Total Time: 40 Minutes

Serves: 12

Ingredients:

- 5 Slices Bacon, Cooked & Crumbled

- 1½ Cups Sour Cream

- 1 Cup Cream Cheese

- 1 Cup Cheddar Cheese, Shredded

- 1 Cup Scallions, Sliced

Directions:

1. Start by heating your oven to 400 degrees F (200 degrees C).

2. Combine all of your ingredients together in a bowl, and then spoon out onto a baking dish.

3. Cook for 25 to 35 minutes. The cheese should be bubbling when it's done.

4. Let it cool slightly before serving.

Nutritional Information:

Total Carbs: 3.5 g

Protein: 6.58 g

Total Fat: 16.76 g

Calories: 190

Supreme Sausage Pizza Bomb

Prep Time: 5-10 Minutes

Total Time: 15-25 Minutes

Serves: 6

Ingredients:

- 12 Italian Sausage Slices

- 8 Black Olives, Pitted

- ¾ Cup Cream Cheese

- 2 Tablespoons Basil, Fresh & Chopped

- 6 Cherry Tomatoes

- Salt to Taste

Directions:

1. Dice your olives and Italian sausage slices.

2. Mix tomatoes, basil and cream cheese together until thoroughly blended.

3. Add your sausage slices and olives into your cream cheese, and then mix thoroughly.

4. Form into balls, and garnish with more basil and olives if desired.

Nutritional Information:

Total Carbs: 1.92 g

Protein: 3.29 g

Total Fat: 11.26 g

Calories: 120

Garlic Coconut Parmesan Chips

Prep Time: 5 Minutes

Total Time: 15-20 Minutes

Serves: 10

Ingredients:

- 1 Cup Parmesan Cheese, Grated

- 4 Tablespoons Coconut Flour

- 1 Teaspoon Rosemary

- ½ Teaspoon Garlic Powder

- ½ Teaspoon Basil

Directions:

1. Start by heating your oven to 350 degrees F (180 degrees C), and then take your Parmesan and flour, mixing it together. Make sure that you use grated Parmesan cheese instead of powdery Parmesan cheese or it'll all start to fall apart.

2. Add your herbs and continue to mix everything together.

3. Line a large baking sheet with parchment paper. Spoon mixture 2 inches apart on prepared baking sheet.

4. Bake for 8-10 minutes or until crisp and golden.

5. Let cool and enjoy!

Nutritional Information

Total Carbs: 1.76 g

Protein: 2.9 g

Total Fat: 2.8 g

Calories: 44

Dijon Mustard Cashew Sausage Ham

Prep Time: 5-10 Minutes

Total Time: 25 Minutes

Serves: 12

Ingredients:

- 3 Slices Pork Ham, Chopped

- 6 Ounces Sausage

- 6 Ounces Cream Cheese, Softened

- ¼ Cup Cashews, Chopped

- 1 Teaspoon Dijon Mustard

Directions:

1. Chop your sausages and pop them in the blender with your cashews, blending until smooth.

2. Beat the cream cheese and mustard together until smooth.

3. Roll your sausage mixture into balls and then form a cream cheese layer over it with your fingers. It should make about twelve balls.

4. Refrigerate them until firm, and then roll each ball in the chopped smoke pork ham before serving.

Nutrition Facts per Serving:

Total Carbs: 3.63 g

Protein: 9.03 g

Total Fat: 12.33 g

Calories: 159

Egg & Cheesy Fat Bombs

Prep Time: 5-10 Minutes

Total Time: 15-20 Minutes

Serves: 6

Nut Free, Sweetener Free

Ingredients:

2 Eggs, Boiled and Chopped

¼ Cup Butter

1 Cup Cream Cheese

½ Cup Blue Cheese, Grated

Directions:

1. Mix cream cheese, grated blue cheese, and butter in a medium mixing bowl.

2. Add in eggs, and continue to stir, making sure it's mixed well.

3. Make six balls, and then place them on parchment paper. Refrigerate for about 2 hours.

Nutritional Information:

Total Carbs: 1.85 g

Protein: 7.65 g

Total Fat: 21.58 g

Calories: 231

Delicious Olive Pesto Bombs

Prep Time: 5 Minutes

Total Time: 15 Minutes

Serves: 4

Ingredients:

- ½ Cup Cream Cheese

- ¼ Cup Pesto Sauce

- 6 Black Olives, Chopped

Directions:

1. Soften your cream cheese slightly, and then add the other two ingredients into the bowl, mixing completely.

2. Pour it into mini muffin cups, and then refrigerate.

Nutritional Information:

Total Carbs: 1.82 grams

Protein: 3.68 grams

Total Fat: 17.7 grams

Calories: 177

Prosciutto Avocado Fat Bombs

Prep Time: 10 Minutes

Total Time: 10 Minutes

Serves: 10

Ingredients:

- 1 Avocado

- 1 Lime

- 10 Slices Prosciutto

Directions:

1. Halve your avocado, remove the seed, and then cut it into large slices.

2. Squeeze lime over avocado slices, and then lay each prosciutto slice on a plate.

3. Place each avocado slice on each prosciutto slice, squeeze a little bit more lime, and roll the prosciutto slice up.

Nutritional Information:

Total Carbs: 2.5 g

Protein: 2.9 gf

Total Fat: 4.5 g

Calories: 60

Cheesy Garlic & Lemon Fat Bombs

Prep Time: 5 Minutes

Total Time: 10 Minutes

Serves: 12

Ingredients:

- ¾ Cup Butter

- 4 Ounces Cream Cheese

- 1½ Lemon

- ¼ Cup Fresh Garlic, Minced

Directions:

1. Soften butter and cream cheese, and then blend them with the lemon juice and garlic. Continue to blend until thoroughly mixed and fluffy.

2. Make small balls using an ice cream scooper on a plate and refrigerate for at least 1 hour before serving.

Nutritional Information:

Total Carbs: 1.68 g

Protein: 1.33 g

Total Fat: 10.45 g

Calories: 105

Thick Cut Bacon Cheese Sticks

Prep Time: 5 Minutes

Total Time: 15 Minutes

Serves: 4

Ingredients:

- 4 Slices Bacon

- 4 Frigo Strings of Cheese (Emmental cheese is a great addition)

Directions:

1. Preheat the oven to 350 degrees F (180 degrees C).

2. Wrap cheese sticks with bacon and secure it together with a toothpick.

3. Bake in the oven for 8-10 minutes.

4. Remove and place on a paper towel to drain while cooling.

Nutritional Information:

Total Carbs: 0.42 g

Protein: 6.86 g

Total Fat: 15.3 g

Calories: 167

Conclusion

Thank you again for buying this book!

I hope you've found this fat bombs Recipes Book helpful, Healthy and delicious, and hopefully after this, you will master your fat bombs technique

If you've enjoyed this book, then I'd like to ask you for a favor, would you be kind enough to leave a review for this book on Amazon? It'd be greatly appreciated!

Thank you and good luck!

Destiny Child

Printed in Great Britain
by Amazon